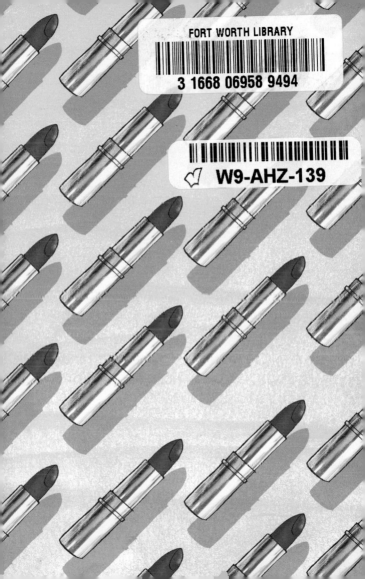

The A to Z of Lipstick

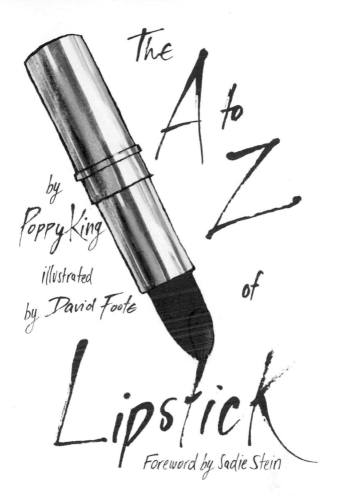

The
A to Z
of
Lipstick

by
Poppy King

illustrated
by David Foote

Foreword by Sadie Stein

ATRIA BOOKS

NEW YORK • LONDON • TORONTO • SYDNEY • NEW DELHI

ATRIA BOOKS
An Imprint of Simon & Schuster, Inc.
1230 Avenue of the Americas
New York, NY 10020

First Atria Books hardcover edition November 2016

ATRIA BOOKS and colophon are trademarks of Simon & Schuster, Inc.

For information about special discounts for bulk purchases,
please contact Simon & Schuster Special Sales at 1-866-506-1949
or business@simonandschuster.com.

The Simon & Schuster Speakers Bureau can bring authors to your
live event. For more information, or to book an event, contact the
Simon & Schuster Speakers Bureau at 1-866-248-3049 or visit our
website at www.simonspeakers.com.

Manufactured in China

10 9 8 7 6 5 4 3 2 1

Library of Congress Cataloging-in-Publication Data

Names: King, Poppy, author.
Title: The A to Z of lipstick / Poppy King ; with illustrations by David Foote.
Description: First Atria paperback edition. | New York : Atria Books, 2017.
Identifiers: LCCN 2016015252 (print) | LCCN 2016019414 (ebook) | ISBN
    9781501141669 (hardback) | ISBN 9781501141683 (eBook)
Subjects: LCSH: Beauty, Personal. | Cosmetics. | Lipstick. | BISAC: HEALTH &
    FITNESS / Beauty & Grooming. | HEALTH & FITNESS / General.
Classification: LCC RA776.98 .K56 2016 (print) | LCC RA776.98 (ebook) | DDC
646.7/26—dc23
LC record available at https://lccn.loc.gov/2016015252

ISBN 978-1-5011-4166-9
ISBN 978-1-5011-4168-3 (ebook)

*This book is dedicated to the
female. To the fascinating, complex,
intriguing, amazing, multitalented,
strong, vulnerable, passionate, driven,
perplexing, awe-inspiring, ever
surprising, incredible female.*

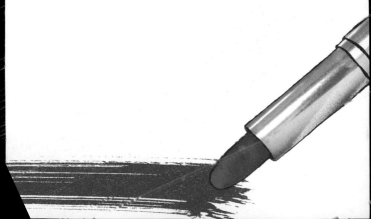

"Be with someone who ruins your lipstick––not your mascara."

—ANONYMOUS

"She has a way with words, red lipstick, and making an entrance."

—Kate Spade

Foreword by Sadie Stein

I remember the first time I saw a Poppy King lipstick. I was fifteen years old, feeling very conspicuous and out of place in Barneys cosmetics department, when there it was: an unintimidating—but alluring—display, in a range of seven enticing shades. This was the '90s, the era of browns and wines, but these lipsticks were different—they were the fresh, bright colors I associated with the wisecracking dames in the old movies I loved. Shyly, feeling clumsy, I tried one on. And there, in the mirror, I saw a vision of the woman I wanted to be: glamorous but assertive, classic but modern. My face looked more alive; I felt visible, but in a way of my choosing. This lipstick didn't seem to have much to do with the glosses and brushes and lip liners I saw in magazines, and which I found so alienating.

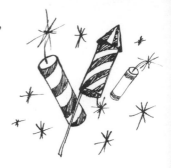

For once, I didn't feel gauche or incompetent or like a fraud—rather, I felt smart, in every way. I felt like me. I'd walked into the store thinking I didn't belong—a bookish, undersized teenager in the wrong kind of clothes—and walked out confident—and incidentally, in possession of my very first red lipstick. It was to be the first of many.

Meeting Poppy herself was a similar experience: here, you recognized at once, was someone who knew who she was. I remember my first sight of her, over breakfast in New York—vibrant, radiating happy energy, and, of course, wearing a bold red lip. I had gotten in touch with her because at that time I had what seemed like a counterintuitive idea: a *Paris Review* lipstick that paid tribute to its early days on the left bank and its early bohemian muses. I was nervous; it seemed like such a long-shot idea—lipstick and a venerable literary magazine— but Poppy was immediately enthusiastic. As a voracious reader, thinker, culture vulture, she got it at once: the inherent glamour of art, and the art of glamour. I was immediately won over by her effervescent charm, too. She went around the SoHo café hugging people she knew and smiling broadly. And her confidence, her enthusiasm, her kindness were all immediately apparent. I knew instinctively that this was someone nourishing—someone who would change my life, again. Incidentally, she had brought Lipstick Queen lipsticks for the waitresses. Poppy is always carrying lipsticks!

Poppy believes deeply in lipstick, and what it can do. When she sees a lipstick, she sees not just pigment and war paint (although she certainly gets that), but history, and empowerment, and self-expression.

She's built a career on making perfectly shaded and formulated lipsticks and showing women how to wear them, but she's been able to do that—and do it again—because she understands that it's more than makeup. Her story is about believing in what you want and going after it fearlessly, and then sharing that message with other women. Poppy sees the potential in the world, which is very different from idealizing it. And she definitely sees the subversive beauty of appropriating makeup for our own empowerment.

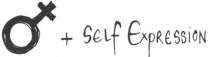 + Self Expression

Poppy has never made as many shades as some of the huge corporate brands. And yet, the funny thing is, her narrower range of colors feels more about self-expression than a shade matched to your skin tone from a thousand choices. In her work around the country and the world, Poppy has met with hundreds of different women—genuinely different—and her lipstick, and her passionate belief in the individual beauty of each person, have allowed her to connect with all of them. They might all be wearing classic red, but in each case it's brought out something particular. Confidence and glamour unite them.

Those two touchstones might be said to guide a lot of Poppy's choices. She's never followed a business rulebook, or anything but her own intuition, and the result has been an array of collaborations and projects that are as idiosyncratic and surprising as they are right: lipsticks dedicated to the 1920s jazz age, to Helmut Newton's 1970s lacquer, to wear with blue jeans. They're all—horrible fashion word—"wearable." And yet each one makes you feel special, daring, a little bold.

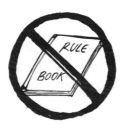

In this book, you'll find Poppy's credo in a nutshell. And like everything she's done, it's also practical: here you'll find not just inspiration but also advice on how to wear lipstick, and how not to be afraid of it. As Poppy explains, the process should be fun and easy and, at the end of the day, look great.

In her words, lipstick "is your passport to glamour . . . and glamour is open to all." And glamour can be as simple—or as complicated—as the perfect shade of red.

———

Sadie Stein is a contributing editor for the Paris Review.

"If eyes are the window of the soul, lips are the mirror of our mood."

—Bobbi Brown

Once upon a time there was a girl who lived in Melbourne, Australia. This was a very little girl who felt very small.

The world seemed like a big, scary place to this little girl. Her father was not well, and passed away when she was seven years of age. This made the little girl very sad.

Her mother was a very stylish lady—a fashion designer who had porcelain skin and hooded green eyes, and wore her hair in a black bob. She wore lovely clothes, with wonderful costume jewelry and fashionable shoes.

She also wore deep bloodred lipstick that she bought from a store across the world called Biba, in London. The little girl loved it when her mother would come home from her overseas trips with a suitcase filled with beautiful and exotic things infused with the sensual musk-and-lilac fragrance.

One day the little girl was playing dress-up—one of her favorite activities—when she sneaked off with one of her mother's lipsticks. Down the long hall to her mother's bedroom she went, holding this precious item.

It was the first time she had ever tried lipstick. She stood in front of her mother's huge wooden dresser. She nervously removed the lid, then wound up the tube, just as she had seen her mother do so many times before.

The little girl knew that putting on lipstick would make her look different on the outside. But what she didn't expect was that the lipstick would make her *feel* so different on the inside. It was like she had put on a superhero cape. Suddenly she felt like a brave, powerful woman and not a tiny little girl.

The lipstick had connected her to a source of strength she didn't know she had. A strength that could transcend anything and enable her to take on the world. It was amazing how that simple swipe of lipstick made her feel. She was entranced with it from that day on.

As the little girl grew up she stopped playing dress-up with her mom's clothes and started exploring her own look. During her teenage years she felt very awkward. She had long, unruly curls and strong features, and was very petite. She didn't look like the other girls she knew. She had a look that was unusual, and she felt unsure of herself.

She tried to fit in and dress like her friends, but it was a strange time in the world—called the '80s—and fashion had taken on all sorts of electric hues, even the lipsticks. The trendy colors were hot pinks and bright oranges, and they didn't suit the teenage girl at all, even though her friends could wear them.

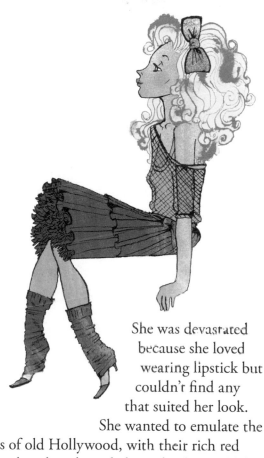

She was devastated
because she loved
wearing lipstick but
couldn't find any
that suited her look.
She wanted to emulate the
stars of old Hollywood, with their rich red
matte lips, but the only lipsticks she could find
were shiny and pink, and many had a frosted
finish that she didn't like. She searched high

and low in department stores and drugstores for 1940s-style lipsticks in deep reds, rusts, and burgundy, but to no avail.

Soon, she was nearing the end of her time in high school, and she was supposed to know what career she wanted to pursue but she had no idea. She once again found herself feeling very unsure of her place in the world.

She still looked for lipsticks that could make her experience the feeling she had the first time she tried her mother's on. Biba had shut down, so now her mother was also searching for bloodred matte lipstick, and together they wondered why they couldn't find it.

One day, after asking yet another salesperson behind the cosmetic counter if she had any lipsticks that were matte and not shiny or shimmery, the woman said, "If I had a dollar for every time someone asked me that, I'd be rich!"

This gave the girl an idea. What if she were to start her own lipstick brand, selling matte, old-Hollywood-style lipsticks? The kind of lipstick she wanted . . . and that apparently other women did too?

Since the girl's father's death, her mother had had to work hard to bring in money for the girl and her brother, so the girl couldn't ask her family for any kind of financial support—and besides she didn't even know how lipstick was even made. But despite this she kept thinking about how to create the lipstick brand of her dreams.

Back in those days, there was no Internet for the girl to turn to—so instead, she turned

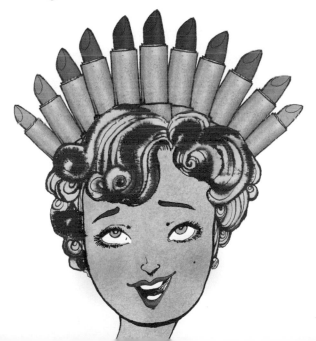

to the phone book. She decided she would look up lipstick factories . . . but she didn't see any of those. What she found instead were listings for cosmetic manufacturers, so she started ringing those and asking if they made lipsticks.

Finally, she found one that did. They said they could make her any type of lipstick she desired—and yes, they could make matte lipsticks—but she had to guarantee a minimum order of a thousand units per shade.

She told them she would come back when she had financing in place, and so she set about looking for ways to raise the money. At eighteen, the girl was not able to get a loan from a bank, so she had to think creatively.

She decided that the best way would be to apply for grants given by the government for small-business start-ups. But to do this, she had to put together a business plan. The girl wasn't sure what that would entail—after all, she was only eighteen and hadn't yet gone to college—so she had to figure it out.

She started asking the advice of anyone

she or her mother knew in the business
world, to see if someone could tell her how to
formulate a business plan. And guess what?
One of the people she went to for advice was
so impressed with her passion for what she was
doing that he decided to become her business
partner, and thus her company was born.

It took the girl just over a year to get
everything ready for launch. She worked with
the factory she had found, showing them
paint chips and fabric swatches as examples of
the colors she wanted in matte lipsticks.

She also found a graphic designer to help
her with the packaging of her lipstick, and
how it would look when displayed in stores.
In March 1992 she was ready with her first
seven lipsticks, which she named after the
Seven Deadly Sins: Lust, Anger, Decadence,
Indolence, Avarice, Envy, and Vanity.

She was enormously proud of her first
few products, but she knew she only had
seven shades. How was she going to get these
noticed among the huge competition from big
brands? She decided that rather than selling

SEVEN DEADLY SINS

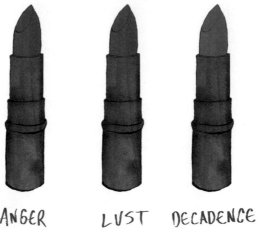

ANGER   LUST   DECADENCE

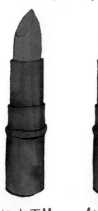 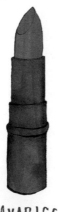 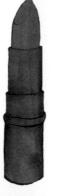 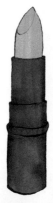

VANITY   AVARICE   ENVY   INDOLENCE

them where women usually bought cosmetics she would approach small fashion boutiques in trendy neighborhoods.

She believed that lipstick should be sold alongside clothing, so she went to one of her favorite stores and asked if they would sell her line. They agreed to give it a chance.

Now that she had a store to sell her lipsticks in, she needed to find a way to promote them. In the front pages of all the glossy magazines are the names of those magazines' beauty editors, so she sent off a box of lipsticks to each of them with a handwritten

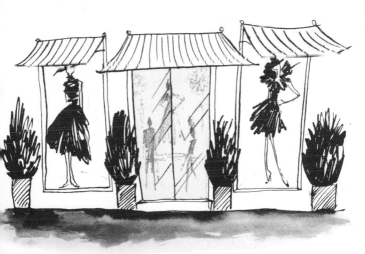

note explaining her brand's creation story: that she couldn't find any lipsticks she liked, so she had decided to start her own company.

Vogue decided to write a small piece, and just like that, the venture took off. More magazines and newspapers became fascinated and wanted to write about this unusual undertaking. At the same time, more stores were asking for the lipsticks and the business started to really grow.

So many people were asking for her lipsticks that she started selling them in big department stores, and by her second year, she had sold more than a million dollars' worth of her product. To celebrate she decided to take herself on a trip to New York City to see what was happening in the rest of the world when it came to cosmetics.

When she arrived in New York she went straight to a wonderful store she had heard about—Barneys. This was a very special store, as it didn't stock the same things that all the other stores sold but looked for unique products from all over the world.

She thought this would be the perfect

place to carry her lipsticks, so she found the phone number of the corporate offices and rang them up. She asked to speak to the cosmetic buyer . . . and to her surprise, she got through.

She told the buyer her story, and that she now had seven shades named after the Seven Deadly Sins. She asked how she might get the chance to meet with a representative from Barneys.

Much to her surprise, yet again, the buyer asked her to come in the next day. Barneys was looking for boutique brands and hers sounded like one they would be interested in. When she presented to them, they loved the entire story, and decided immediately that they would feature the lipsticks in the brand-new store they were opening on Madison Avenue.

When the Seven Deadly Sins finally launched in New York, it was to great success. Lines of people arrived at the counter, asking for the lipsticks they had been reading about in the press.

All the while, the business was continuing to grow in Australia. The girl brought out more shades and the brand developed a cult following. News was spreading to other countries as well, but keeping up with demand in Australia was hard enough.

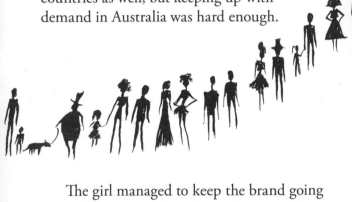

The girl managed to keep the brand going strong for six years, but she ran into trouble trying to expand. She had taken on some partners to help her with the needs of the growing business, but the fit was not great. They had very different ideas as to how things should be done, and ultimately, she had to sell to new partners in order to keep the business going. She remained CEO of the brand, but she no longer owned it, so she took a backseat in the running of the company.

The brand continued to grow for another four years, but it was never the same, and she wondered about the next phase of her life. She was now turning thirty and was ready for new challenges. It wasn't long before an opportunity came to her.

She was contacted by one of the biggest cosmetics companies in the world, which asked if she would be interested in moving to New York and coming up with product ideas for one of their brands. She decided to take the position. She packed up all her things and headed to New York City, ready for her new life.

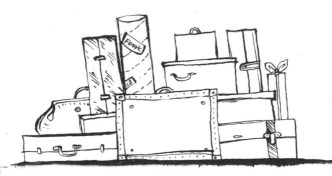

But as much as she thrived on the new adventure that the Big Apple provided, she had been an entrepreneur ever since she finished high school, and she didn't mesh in the corporate world. She lasted in the job for three years. In that time, she had fallen in love with her new home, and decided to stay on in New York.

She wanted to return to her true passion— creating lipsticks and running her own brand. She decided to start her own company again, but this time, with all the knowledge she had gained from her previous experiences, plus all she had learned while working for a big corporation.

Lipstick Queen was launched, and once again, she was in charge of a brand entirely focused on lipstick! It was 2006, and many women were wearing lip gloss instead of lipstick. She wanted to advocate the wonders of lipstick so it didn't end up going the way of the dinosaur.

Her brand returned to Barneys, where it is to this day; it is also sold in many other stores around the world. In the many years since, that grown-up little girl has spoken to thousands of other women about their hopes, dreams, and desires around lipstick.

Yes, the little girl who fell in love with lipstick when she was playing dress-up is me,

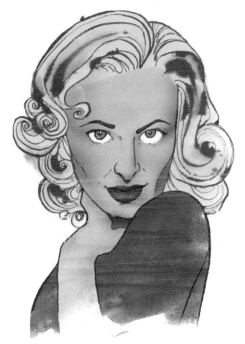

Poppy King, cosmetics entrepreneur and passionate devotee of the magical powers of lipstick.

For more than twenty-five years now I have been creating, designing, developing, wearing, and loving lipstick.

Lipstick is more than a cosmetic. Cosmetics conceal, correct, or enhance, but only lipstick *transforms*. It transforms your sense of self and what you believe is possible. It is your passport to glamour . . . and glamour is open to all.

No matter her age, size, or income, any woman can be glamorous. Unlike beauty, which is apparent in a set of physical features, glamour comes from a mind-body connection. Glamour is about your feminine spirit, and the fastest way I know to connect to that spirit is through lipstick.

The magic of lipstick is what happens on the inside when you wear it, which then manifests on the outside. You are capable of anything with your lipstick on. Yet despite this, so many women are confused and unsure of which lipstick to wear and fearful that it will become a high-maintenance habit.

The simple fact is, all women can wear lipstick without difficulty. This little book will

tell you everything you've wanted to know
about this fascinating product. From how
to find what suits you and how a lipstick is
developed, to what certain colors say about
you, and everything in between.

After all, lipstick tells a story. It tells the
world you are here and ready to participate in
all it has to offer.

Many of us feel a deep, emotional
connection to lipstick, more so than to any other
makeup we might wear. I have often said that
lipstick is to women what a sports car is to men,
something that all women are mesmerized by
but not all believe they can pull off.

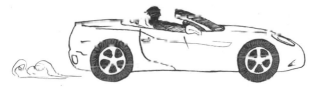

I'm here to tell you that you can, and this
book will show you how.

Through all the ups and downs I have
been through, all the triumphs and all
the failures, all the dreams and all the
disappointments, lipstick has remained my

constant. I return to it day after day as a source of enchantment and strength. And all those years ago, when I swiped that red across my lips, I could never have foreseen the adventures it has taken me on.

Now it's time for your lipstick story to begin. You never know what can happen, what amazing opportunities are out there until you try—one lipstick at a time.

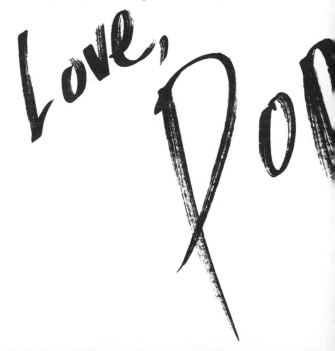

Love, Po

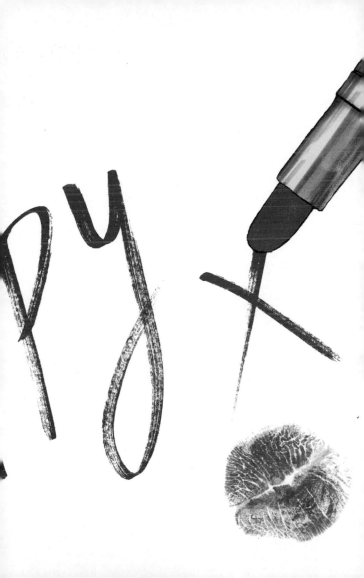

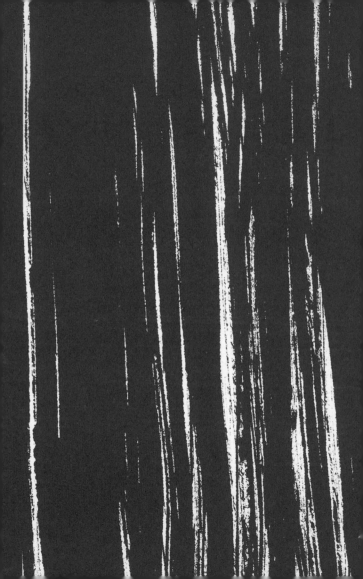

"Treat your makeup like jewelry for the face. Play with colors, shapes, structure—it can transform you."

—François Nars

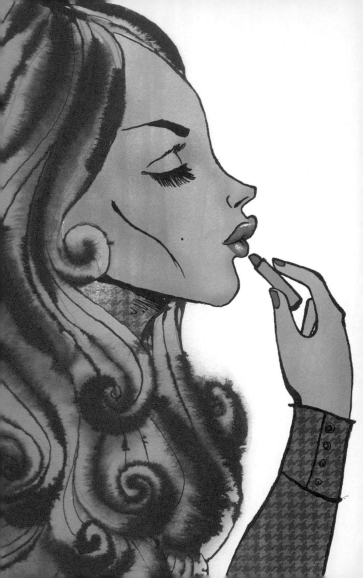

A is for APPLY

Forget all the rules you have heard about how to apply lipstick. Using it straight from the tube is the best way to get the full effect of the color. You can use a lip liner if you are worried about the edges and a lip brush if you want to sheer it out, but a good lipstick can always go straight from the tube to the lip.

> *Lip tip:* If you find yourself going through multiple steps in applying a lipstick, then it may not be the right formula for you—lipstick should be easy!

EASY STEP-BY STEP LIPSTICK APPLICATION

1. Apply lipstick straight from the tube if you want full pigment
2. Blot first coat with a tissue to make the base long-lasting
3. Apply an additional top coat and . . . voilà!

By using this application method, you should only need to touch up a few times a day, usually after eating.

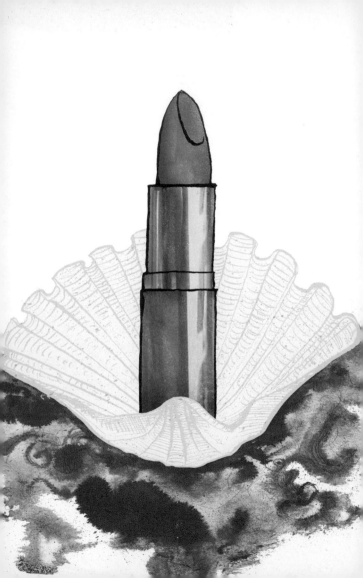

B is for BREAK FREE

Many women love the idea of lipstick but are afraid to wear it. Don't be! But before you try lipstick, get ready to think about yourself differently. Over time we build up an idea of ourselves that feels set in stone. It's not! Lipstick helps you challenge the assumptions you have made about yourself. Break out of your shell with a fiery red or luscious pink lip color.

Lip tip: We all get stuck in ruts—emotionally, psychologically, even stylistically. Lipstick is one of the easiest and most cost-effective ways of escaping that rut.

C is for CREAM

Cream lipstick (sometimes packaged as "satin") is moisturizing, and a perfect choice for dry, cracked lips. It's not as long-lasting as some other formulas, however, so be prepared to reapply throughout the day.

Lip tip: To make a cream lipstick last longer, be sure to blot your lips and apply a second coat.

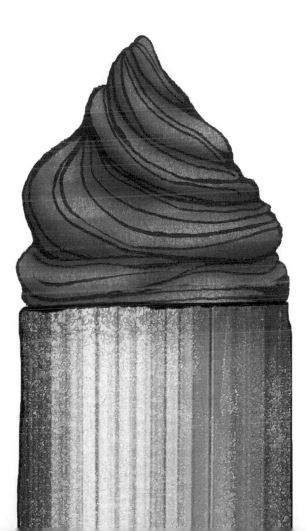

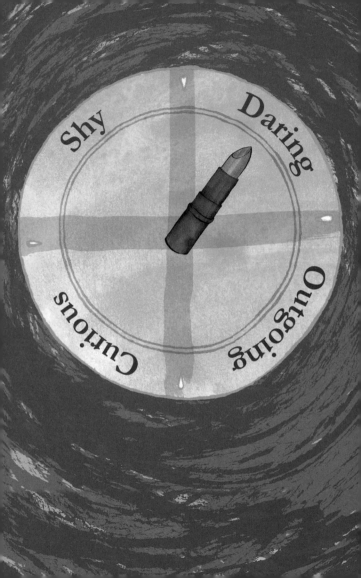

D is for DARING

Turn your confidence up. It's easy to think that you have to be daring to wear lipstick, when actually, it's the other way around—wearing lipstick makes you *feel* daring. It's an instant confidence booster.

Lip tip: Studies have shown that women who wear lipstick smile more often

E is for EXPERIMENT

Lipstick is supposed to be fun! Experiment with colors and formulas. You don't need any special knowledge to know how to find a lipstick for you. You just need the willingness to try. Soon, you will start learning what works for you and what doesn't.

Lip tip: Remember that lipstick is not a tattoo—it is easily removed, so go ahead and play with as many as you can.

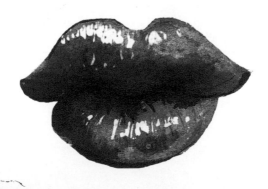

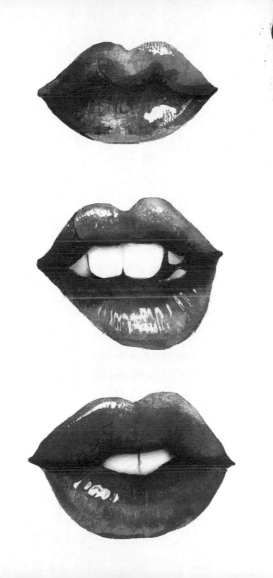

"Where lipstick is concerned, the important thing is not the color but to accept God's final word on where your lips end."

—Jerry Seinfeld

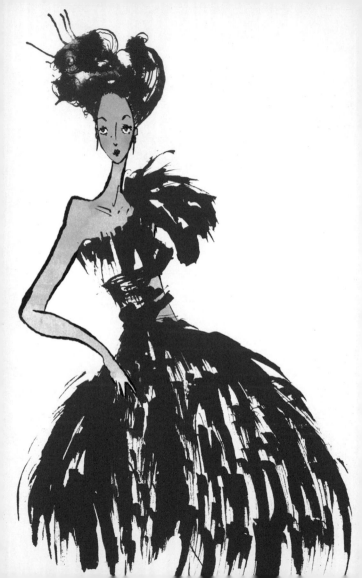

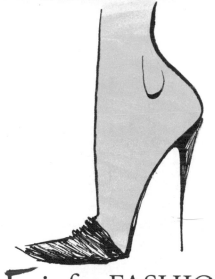

F is for FASHION

It can be hard to keep up with fashion trends that change every season. Instead of changing your wardrobe, try changing your lip color. With a new lipstick, your whole wardrobe seems fresh again. Clothes you have worn for years are suddenly exciting with a different lip shade.

Lip tip: Try on the same outfits with and without lipstick and you will learn to see the difference it can have on your overall sense of style.

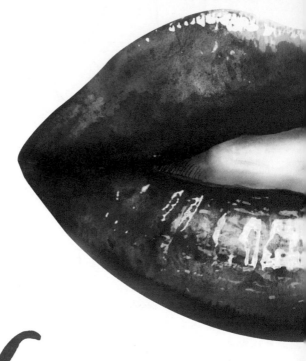

G is for GLOSSY

Glossy lipsticks give your lips a shiny, sparkling finish. But these formulas are more likely to bleed. Be sure to blot delicately after application.

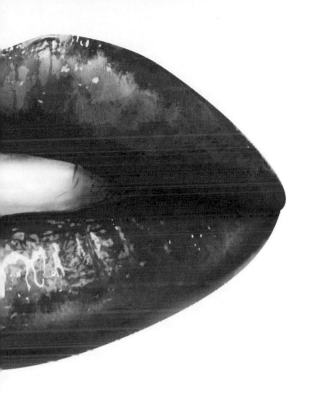

{ *Lip tip:* Use some under-eye concealer around the edges of your lips to prevent bleeding or feathering.

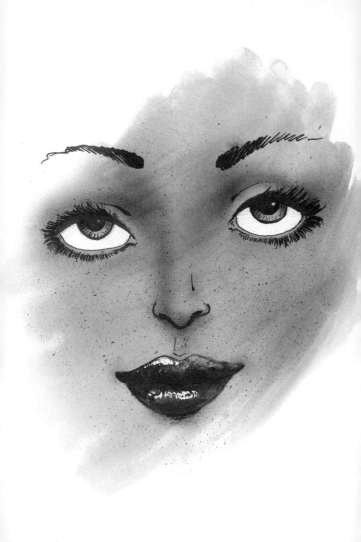

H is for HIGHLIGHT

Let your lipstick highlight your face.
Don't think of it as something that has to
accompany a full face of makeup (especially
eye makeup). Lipstick looks incredibly fresh
and extremely modern when worn with
minimal other cosmetics.

Lip tip: Try putting on your
lipstick before you do your eye
makeup. This will help you assess how
much is too much far more easily.

"Hand me my purse, will you darling? A girl can't read that sort of thing without her lipstick."

—Audrey Hepburn, *Breakfast at Tiffany's*

HISTORY of lipstick

The art of painting the lips dates all the way back to ancient times where it was done as part of rituals and to honor the gods. Lipstick first appeared as a symbol of glamour in Egypt with Cleopatra, who became famous not just for her dark kohl eye makeup but for her ruby-red lips painted with rouge made with carmine (a pigment derived from an insect called the cochineal). Carmine is used in lipstick to this day.

It became very aspirational to paint the lips red, but with the fall of the Egyptian empire and the rise of the Dark and Middle Ages in Europe, the Catholic Church took over as the ultimate dictator of acceptable fashion and grooming practices. Lip color was associated with Satan and therefore relegated to the very bottom of the social ladder.

There it remained until the late sixteenth century, when Queen Elizabeth I brought it back into vogue, with her stark white makeup and crimson lip stain made from beeswax and

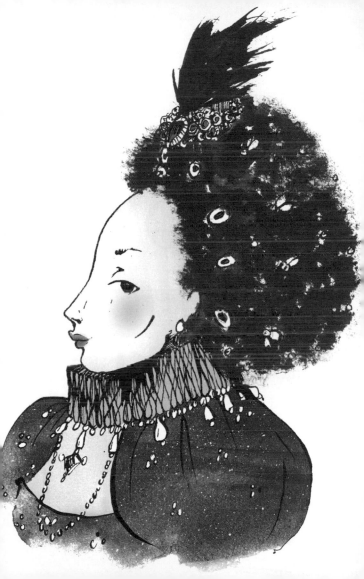

red plants. Like Cleopatra before her, Elizabeth elevated lip coloring, and soon many high-class women sought to imitate her style.

After Elizabeth's death, lipstick slipped from fashion, and until the late nineteenth century lip coloring remained a practice reserved for performers and prostitutes.

But by the end of the nineteenth century, the rise of industrialization had allowed lipstick to be mass-produced, and its usage started to spread again. In 1884 the French cosmetic company Guerlain created the first commercial lipstick. They made it from deer tallow, castor oil, and beeswax, and then covered it in silk paper. Lipstick did not yet come in a tube, but came in small pots, and was applied with a fine brush.

Around this time, famous French actress Sarah Bernhardt began wearing lipstick in public—and by 1912, fashionable American women were using lipstick as an important part of their daily beauty regimen. In 1915

Maurice Levy invented the cylindrical metal containers that hold lipstick today, but it wasn't until 1923 that the swivel-up tube was patented by James Bruce Mason Jr. in Nashville, making lipstick much easier to apply.

The 1920s saw a rise in photography and cinema, which made movie stars fashion icons—and their lipstick was sought after. In the 1930s the cosmetics company Max Factor capitalized on the growing mystique around film stars and started replicating the products that were worn onscreen, including lipsticks.

During World War II, lipstick became scarce due to rationing, yet wearing it was also considered patriotic, as it denoted optimism and strength in a time of hardship.

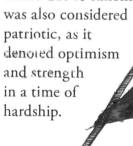

This was thanks to Rosie the Riveter, the famous depiction of a female factory worker with red lips doing the work that was needed while men were away at war. She became a symbol of carrying on in good faith.

By the 1950s, movie star glamour was in full effect, with stars such as Marilyn Monroe and Elizabeth Taylor sporting dark red lips and popularizing them for the masses.

With the 1960s and the rise of rock and roll came dramatic new ideas in fashion, as well as lipstick. Anything went—from pastel shades to white and silver. By the late '60s and '70s, however, lipstick had lost some popularity, as the hippie trend took over, and a more natural look came into favor.

Lipstick returned with a vengeance in the 1980s with the rise of the power woman and her bulletproof shoulder pads. Lip colors were bright and garish—mostly hot pink and fuchsia. The 1990s and the emerging grunge trends saw a backlash to this, with browns and deep hues coming into fashion.

By the early 2000s, lipstick had taken a

backseat to lip gloss, which was considered a fuss-free alternative. These days, however, we are seeing a renewed interest in lipstick—not as a makeup "must-have" but as a personal fashion choice. Major cosmetics houses are revamping their lines, releasing new lipstick formulas, which contain varied ingredients and allow for a vast array of finishes.

Lipstick remains one of the world's simplest and most glamorous products. And its application is one of the few grooming rituals that connect us back through centuries to the experience of being female. In any given age, lipstick—its presence or absence—tells us something about the world we are living in and the hopes and dreams of the era. It is a true cultural barometer—one that measures not just the state of fashion but that of the psyche.

"Pour yourself a drink, put on some lipstick, and pull yourself together."

—Elizabeth Taylor

A LOOK AT LIPSTICK
Through the
Twentieth Century

1920s:

The flappers wore deep wine, almost black lipstick, which symbolized their sexual emancipation. These were the original *Sex and the City* gals—dancing all night and bed-hopping with their bobbed hair and dark lips.

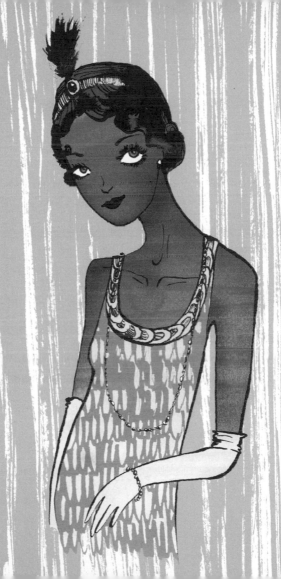

1930s:

During the Great Depression, lipstick sales actually rose as women looked for little luxuries to keep their spirits up. It was from here that the term *lipstick index* arose, which has shown time and time again that when the stock market is down, lipstick sales rise.

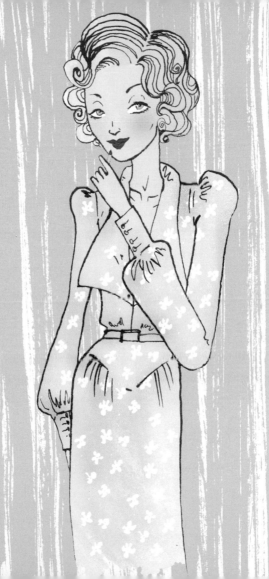

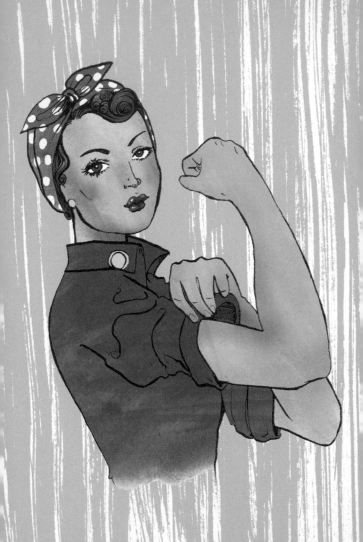

1940s:

WWII descends, and red lipstick becomes a symbol of patriotism and dedication to the war effort.

1950s:

With a return to peacetime and a focus on the home, lipstick colors became very soft and feminine, with pink, coral, and rose-hued tones signifying domestic harmony.

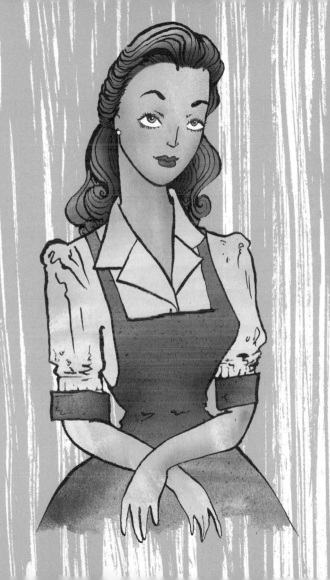

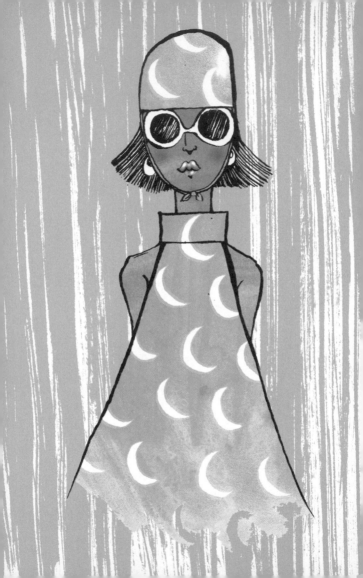

1960s:

The "youthquake" and the rise of hippie culture saw all manner of crazy colored lipsticks, mainly in very white-based pastel tones and even silver, which also reflected the Space Race that defined the decade.

1970s:

Continuing to break from convention, the '70s saw a move away from lipstick to a natural look, with lip gloss coming into fashion, along with increasing sexual freedom.

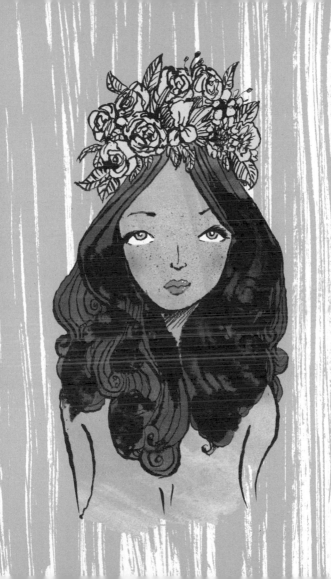

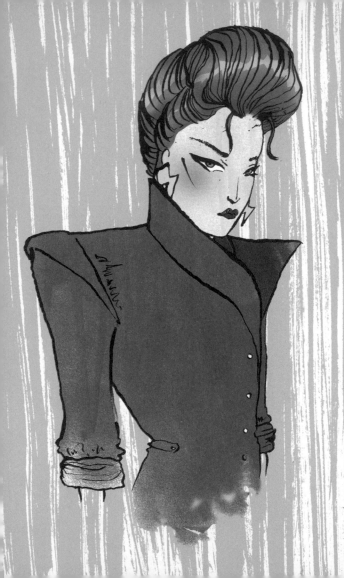

1980s:

The rise of the Power Woman leads to a sudden return to a full face of makeup in bright, bold colors. The new female executive look was part boardroom and part war room—with the war paint to match.

1990s:

The rainbow colors of the '80s deepen to
matte browns and rusty reds with the growing
devotion to grunge.

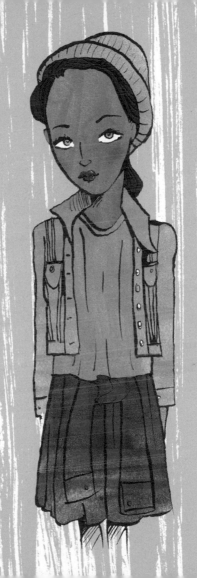

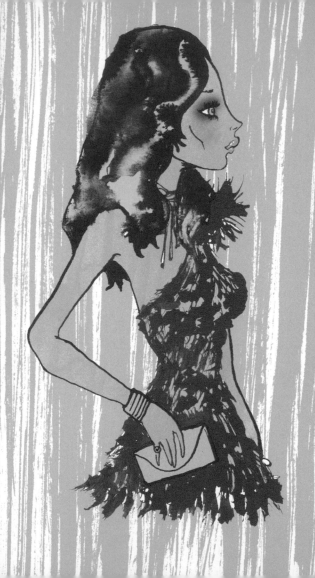

2000s:

The rise of the smoky eye and nude, glossy lips
is seen as the epitome of glamour.

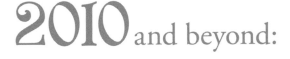

2010 and beyond:

The pendulum swings again—once the dark eye and pale lip become normalized, vibrant lip color reemerges as a way to differentiate from this look.

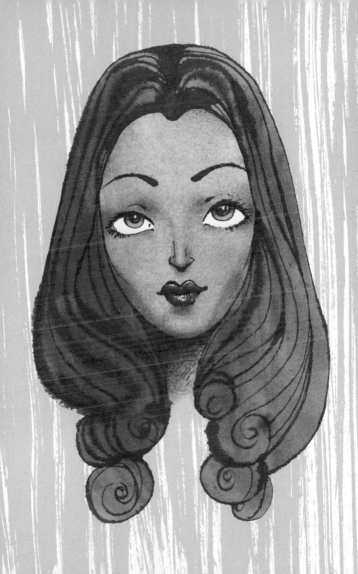

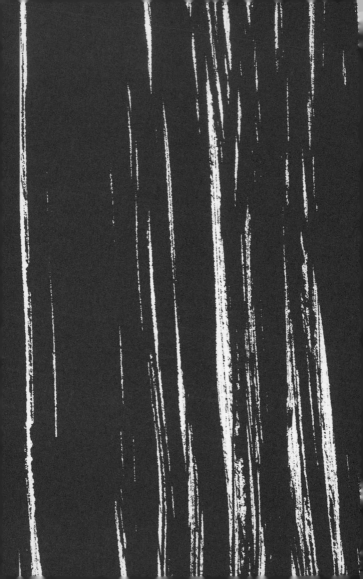

"Beauty to me is about being comfortable in your own skin. That or a kick-ass red lipstick."

—Gwyneth Paltrow

HOW is lipstick made?

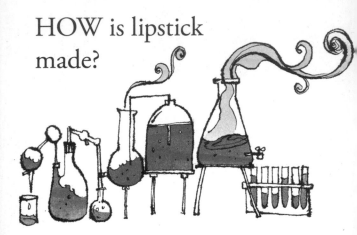

All lipstick is made from the same basic ingredients—however, it is the variations in the quality of these ingredients, as well as the ratios in which they're used, that result in the different products you see on the market.

The basic ingredients fall into three general categories: oils, waxes, and pigments. It is the relationship among these that affects the final result. For example, a lipstick with more pigment than oils is going to be more opaque and more matte, whereas a lipstick with a higher oil content will be shinier.

From idea to reality

1. Ideation: To create any product, the entrepreneur must begin with a concept. For lipstick, the ideation stage involves a marketer determining how she or he wants a new product to feel on the lips or developing a particular marketing approach. In my case, my concept was matte lipstick, named after the seven deadly sins.

2. Formulation: The marketer then briefs the chemist on what attributes and shades she or he is looking for, and the chemist comes up with a formula that best fits the brief.

3. Sampling: Samples are given to the marketer for she or he to evaluate how well the product represents the original concept presented. Tweaks are then made to the formulation. For example, if a lipstick is too sheer, more pigment is added in; if the formulation is too cakey, then the formula is based out (more oil is added to make it lighter).

4. Testing: Once a submission from the lab bench has been approved, the lipstick then goes into testing for stability to ensure the

formula is chemically stable and can be scaled up—meaning produced in quantities that will yield many thousands of lipsticks—and still remain constant.

5. Production: Lipstick in liquid form is formulated in giant vats and then poured into molds that resemble bullets. These are either hand placed or machine placed into what is called the primary packaging, the actual lipstick tube.

6. Packaging: The tubes of lipstick are then packed into what is called the secondary packaging, for those lipsticks that come in boxes.

7. Pack-out: The boxed lipsticks are then packed into shipping containers and are ready to be distributed to stores.

Creating a lipstick from scratch is like testing any other kind of recipe. You think of a dish you want to eat and develop a recipe. You taste it as you're cooking and note whether it needs more salt, whether the consistency is too thick or thin. Any variations in the details make one recipe different from the next.

IDEAS for lipsticks

All makeup manufacturers have different ways
in which they come up with lipsticks. Some of
us are inspired by an ingredient, such as shea
butter, and decide that we want to make a
buttery lipstick. Some of us are first inspired by
a concept and then create a lipstick that reflects
it. For example, one of my lipsticks is called
Velvet Rope. I wanted to create a premium
lipstick—one that gave the wearer a feeling she
was going behind the velvet rope, into the VIP
section—that had a luxe, velvety finish. Either
approach can lead to a beautiful product.

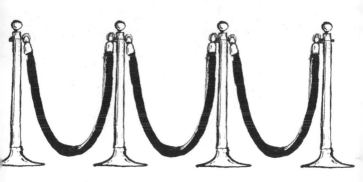

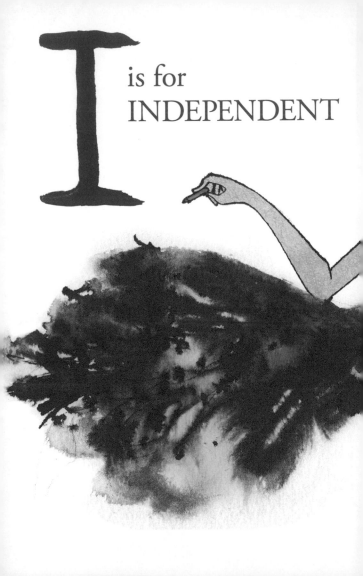

I is for
INDEPENDENT

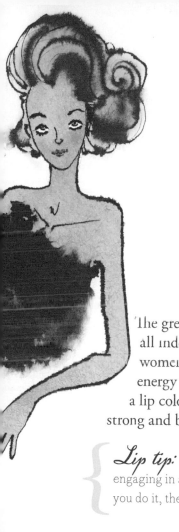

The great lipstick icons were all independent, trailblazing women. Tap into that female energy and power by wearing a lip color that makes you feel strong and brave.

{ *Lip tip:* Wearing lipstick is like engaging in any other habit—the more you do it, the more natural it feels.

ICONS OF LIPSTICKS
Through the Years

Cleopatra: Cleopatra was the original glamour queen. She was well known for her dramatic eye makeup, but the ancient Egyptian ruler was also a fan of dark lips. It was during her reign (51–12 BCE) that the art of painting one's lips became recognized as something that required precision and technique. After all, looking your best was very important to Cleopatra. An icon of seduction, she loved bling and was not afraid to show it.

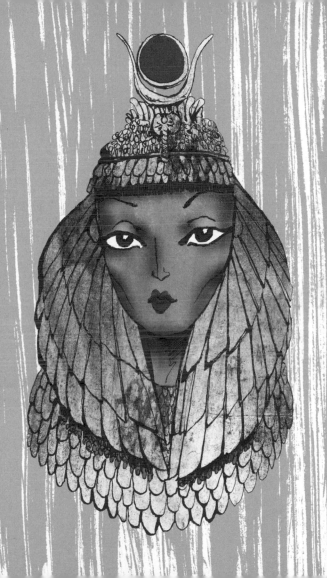

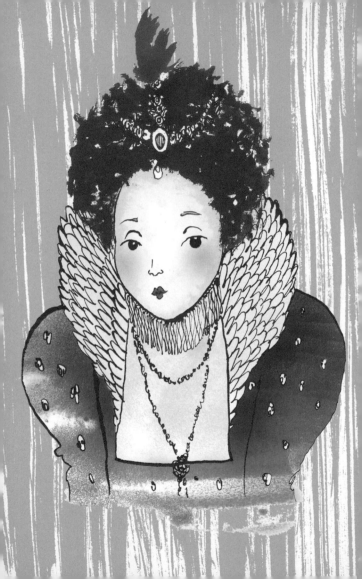

Elizabeth I: During the reign of Elizabeth I (1558–1603) it became fashionable again to wear lipstick. The queen's iconic pale skin contrasted with vibrant colors on the lips was the "In" look of the time. During the medieval years, lipstick was considered sinful, but now that their queen wore it with pride, women everywhere sought out cosmetic vendors on the street to re-create her style. Without Elizabeth I, lipstick may have stayed in the dark ages.

Clara Bow: Her films may have been silent, but her lips were anything but. Clara Bow was one of the first true movie stars of the 1920s, an era when films were becoming the great influencers of fashion and makeup. She became an icon for her "Cupid's bow": dark, perfectly etched-out lips with an exaggerated lip line that really worked for the black-and-white films of the day.

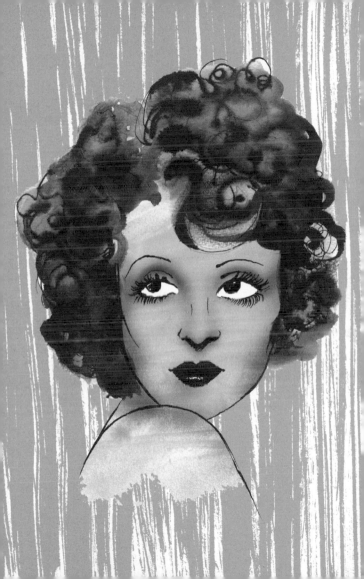

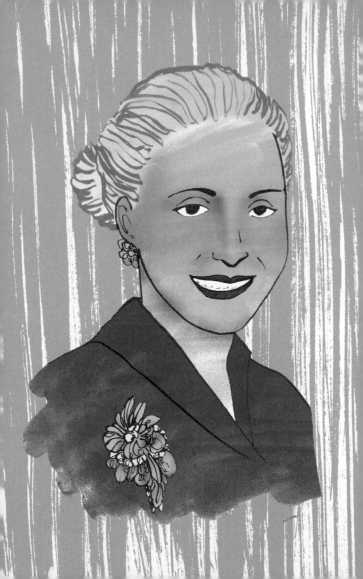

Evita: Eva Perón (Evita) was the First
Lady of Argentina and a real-life Cinderella,
coming from humble beginnings to marry
Argentine president Juan Perón in 1945. She
also became a style icon and was never seen
without her red lips. She brought glamour to
politics and has become synonymous with
female power. Evita was a passionate woman
who fought for women's rights, and today she
remains an icon of style and substance.

Marilyn Monroe: The ultimate femme fatale, no one has elevated red lipstick more than Marilyn Monroe. With her bombshell looks and seductive voice she put the va-va-voom into lipstick, making it playful, sexy, and a must-have for the alluring female. Before Marilyn, red lipstick was simply a shade—she made it a statement. Marilyn and her bright-lipped smile are iconic.

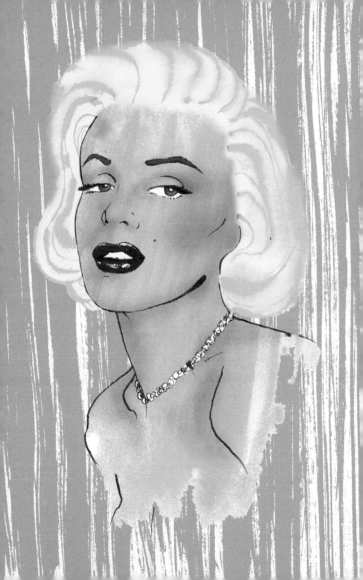

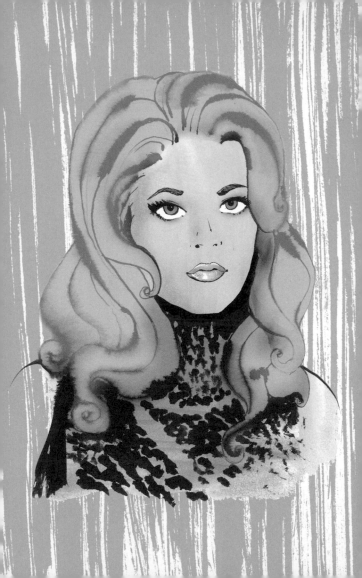

Jane Fonda: Jane Fonda as Barbarella in the 1968 film brought sci-fi to lipstick. The pale, metallic, space-age lip colors she wore on screen were perfect for the time, and Barbarella became an icon of the space race, which defined the latter part of the sixties. She put the sex kitten in outer space with far-out colors that spoke to a new generation.

Andy Warhol: Andy Warhol

elevated lips to an art form: whether it was his iconic portraits of women, among them Elizabeth Taylor, Marilyn Monroe, Audrey Hepburn, and Jackie Kennedy, where red lips were front and center, or his paintings of simply lips themselves. Like the Campbell's soup can, Warhol made lipstick an essential element of pop art, taking it to a level of iconography that was associated with irreverence and fun. Lipstick goes pop thanks to him!

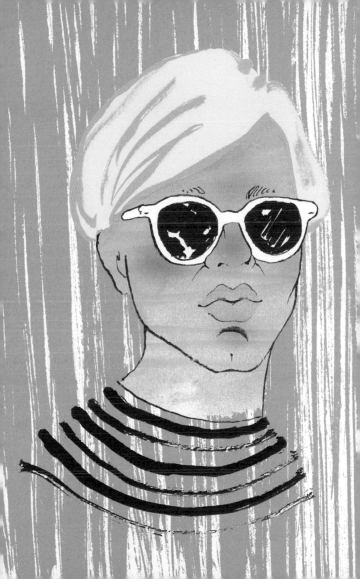

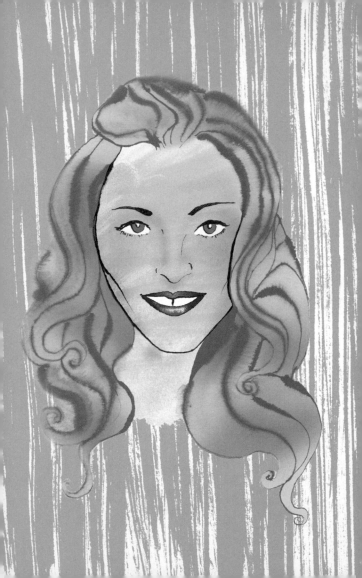

Madonna:

Madonna defined a new era of girl power with her black lace bodysuits and crimson lips. She ushered red lipstick back in as a symbol of strength and moxie, and she turned fashion on its head by making underwear outerwear. Her lipstick became a symbol for glamorous rebellion, and an essential for bad girls looking to have a good time. She was the icon of how nice it is to be naughty, and, to this day, nothing says that more than a strong red lip.

Uma Thurman: Thurman in the cult classic *Pulp Fiction* was the icon of '90s lip glamour with her vamp dark lipstick shade and black bob hair-do. At a time when grunge dominated the fashion world, she injected elegance with attitude into the movement with her lipstick, and exemplified the transformative power of a great lip color.

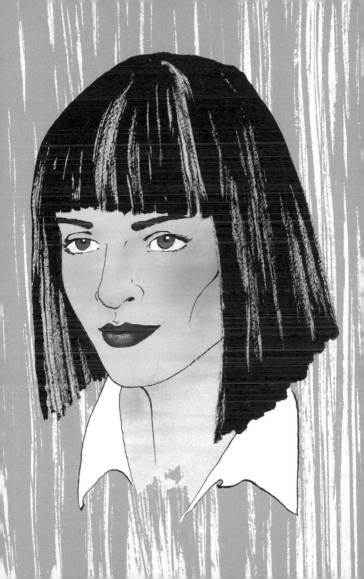

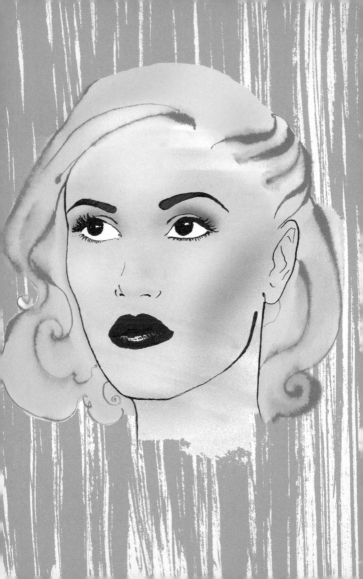

Gwen Stefani: The ultimate

rock chick bringing street cred to red lipstick, Gwen Stefani is an icon of tough girl glamour. No matter what era she's channeling in her fashion, her red lips are always present. She juxtaposes red lipstick and edginess and rocks out with class and just enough defiance. She shows us how to be a rebel while still being über feminine.

Lady Gaga: Challenging beauty conventions on every level—whether it be wearing a dress made of meat or arriving to an event in an egg—Lady Gaga is the icon of extremes. Especially when it comes to her makeup: whether they're red, nude, or purple, Lady Gaga makes a statement with her lips and goes where others fear to tread. Fierce and fabulous, her lipstick is always an essential piece of her performance art.

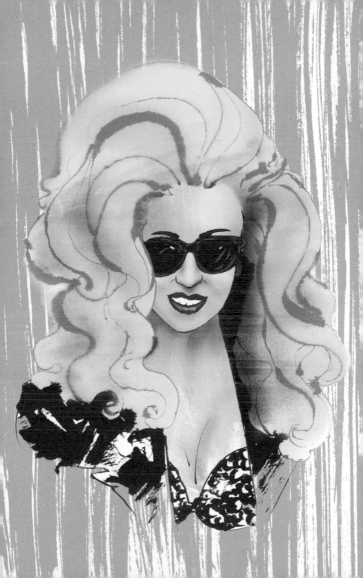

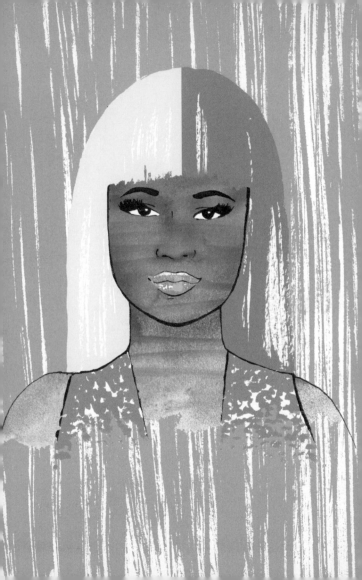

Nicky Minaj:

Just when you thought bubble gum colors on the lips could never be in vogue again, then comes rapper Nicki Minaj to prove you wrong. Known for defying stereotypes in her music and fashion, Nicki has elevated bright lip shades, and in doing so, she reminds us to have fun being female.

Taylor Swift:

Fresh-faced and yet sophisticated, Taylor Swift is rarely seen without her red lips. She has shown women everywhere how to make red lipstick young and modern by wearing it with minimal makeup. She has become a glamour icon for today by taking the best of other eras and mixing them with her own unique sensibility and no-muss, no-fuss attitude. Thanks to Taylor, a new generation of young women now know how chic red lipstick is when worn without a full face of makeup.

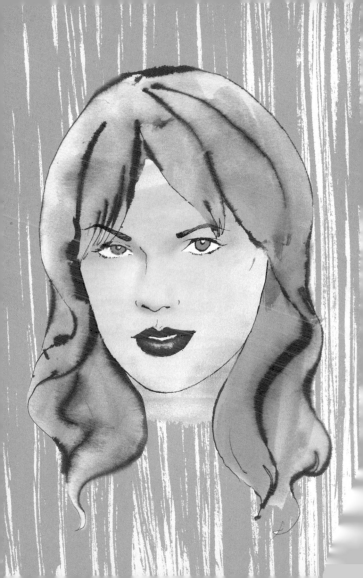

"She was the kind of girl who wore dark lipstick and didn't need to speak a word to seduce you."

—Stephen F. Campbell

J is for JEWELRY

With lipstick on, you may not need as much jewelry as you're used to. Lipstick can make a real statement, so go lighter on your accessories to keep your look clean and polished.

Lip tip: When wearing lipstick, especially bolder colors, think either earrings or a necklace—but rarely both.

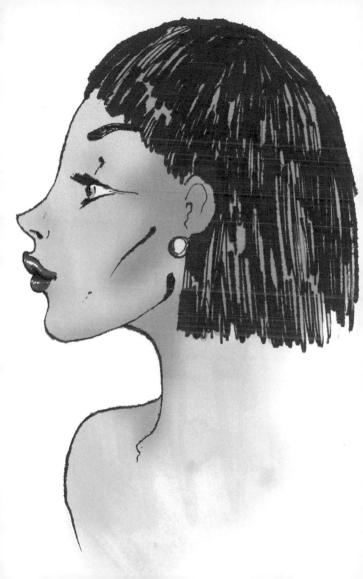

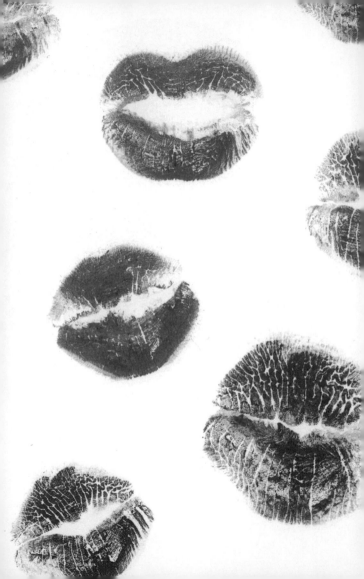

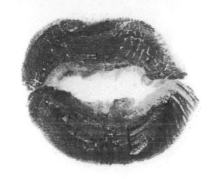

K is for KISSABLE

Lush lip color makes you look even more kissable!

{ *Lip tip:* For the ultimate in kissable color, go with rosebud shades.

L is for LIGHTS UP

A lipstick that suits you will light up your hair, skin, and eyes immediately. You will see those three features brighten as though a light switch went on inside you. Ones that don't suit you as well will not give this light-up effect. After trying multiple lipsticks, you'll soon see the difference between those that light you up and those that don't.

Lip tip: Make sure to look in a full-length mirror as well as the usual handheld mirrors at counters to decide whether a certain hue works for you. After all, lipstick affects not just your face, but your whole look. When you see yourself in a full-length mirror, you will see the lipstick in the entire context of your outfit.

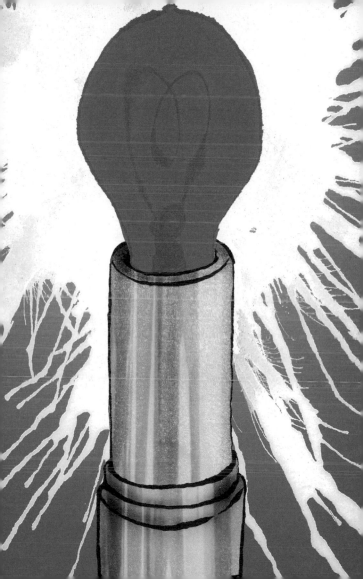

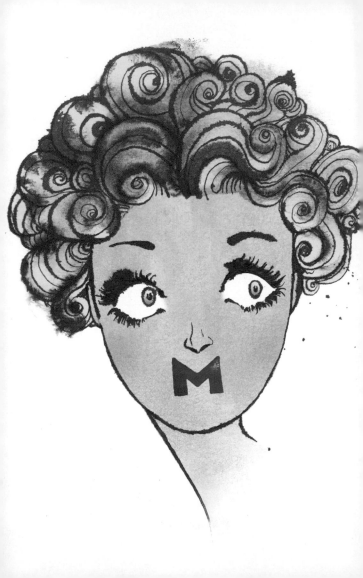

M is for MATTE

Matte lipsticks (my personal favorite!) are long-lasting and often intense in hue.

Lip tip: Matte lipsticks can be drier than other formulas, so be sure to apply some lip balm first.

N is for NAILS

Matching your nail color to your lip shade is the ultimate in glamour, but it's also fun to mix it up and do the opposite. A bold lip with a subtle nail hue or the other way around is a beautiful, wearable look.

Lip tip: The matchy-matchy look works best when you really commit to it. Don't be afraid to go super bold with lip and nail color—just pare back the rest of your makeup.

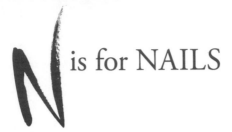

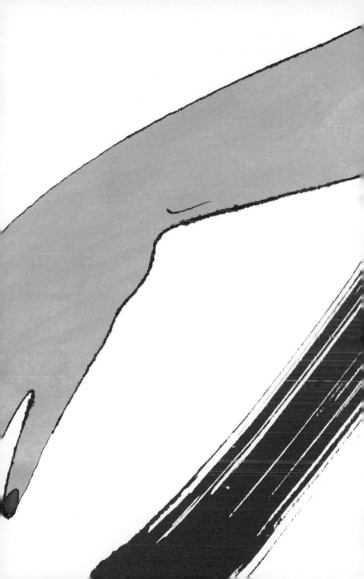

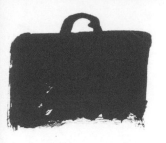

WORK

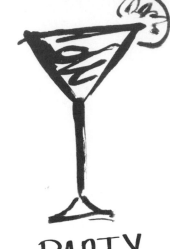

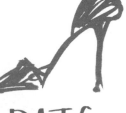

DATE

PARTY

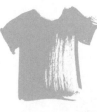

CASUAL

FORMAL

O is for OCCASIONS

Which lip colors work best for which occasions?

Work: Berries, pinky nudes, deep reds

Party: Pinks, wines, bright reds

Date: Rose, nudes, sheer reds

Casual: Nudes, corals, dusty pinks

Formal: Deep wines, reds, pinks

Lip tip: Don't wait for a big occasion to test out a new lipstick. Try wearing it around the house to "break it in," the way you would a new pair of shoes. It's important to bond with a new lipstick shade and let it become part of you.

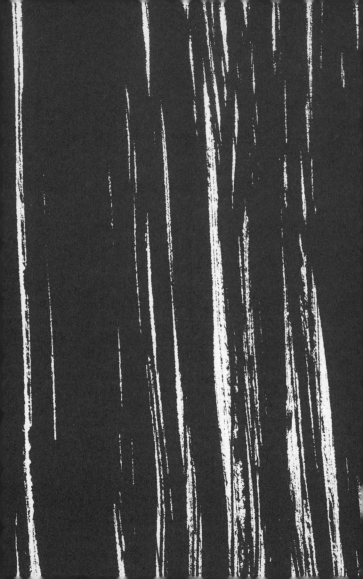

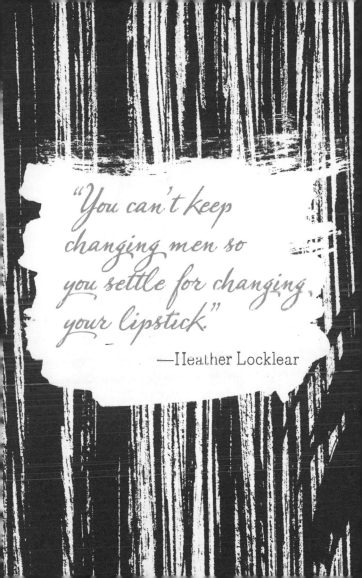

"You can't keep changing men so you settle for changing your lipstick."

—Heather Locklear

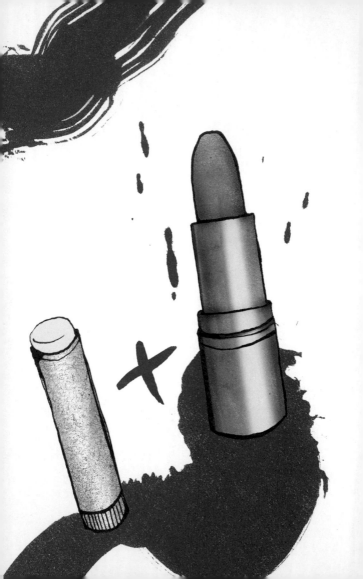

P is for PREP

It's easy to prep your lips for lipstick. If you have dry lips, apply some lip balm first for a moisturizing effect. Look for a lip balm that isn't too glossy so it doesn't alter the texture of your lipstick. If you're worried about bleeding or feathering, use a lip liner.

Lip tip: You can use lip liner before or after applying lipstick. If you've never used it before, it's easier to add it at the end, just to fill in the edges.

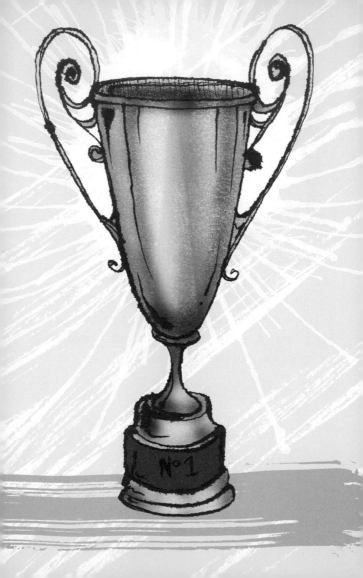

Q is for QUALITY

Quality matters with lipstick. A good-quality product features ingredients like shea butter that keep your lips in good condition and don't dehydrate them.

Lip tip: Any lipstick that requires too many steps is not the right the lipstick for you.

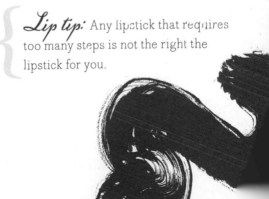

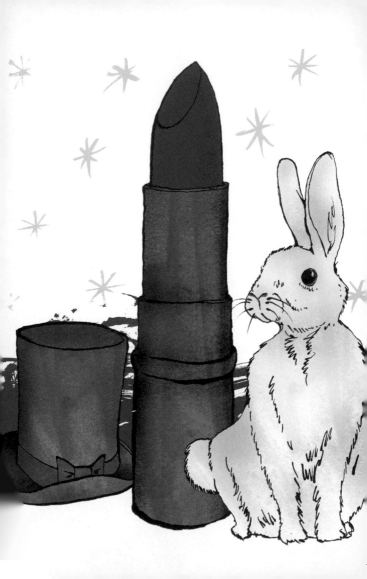

R is for RED

Red lipstick is simply magic! While there are many beautiful shades of lipstick, red lipstick is still the most iconic, and as a result, it has the power to totally transform your mood and make you feel capable of anything. Every woman can wear red lipstick—you don't have to be a movie star to pull it off! We all have red tones naturally occurring in our lips, so it's impossible for it not to look good.

Lip tip: If you're hesitant, try a sheer red first, to allow yourself to get used to seeing yourself in red lipstick.

Guide to COLORS

Generally, the fairer your hair and skin, the more warm, or yellow-based, colors suit you. The darker your hair and skin, the more cool, or blue-based, colors suit you.

> *Lip tip:* How can you tell the difference between warm and cool colors? Warm colors tend toward red, orange, and yellow. Cool colors tend toward pink and purple. Think of the beach: The sand is warm and yellow, and the sea is cool and blue.

COLOR CHART

What do these lip colors say about you?

Pink: **Flirty**

Red: **Glamorous**

Nude: **Subtle**

Orange: **Fun**

Wine: **Intriguing**

Coral: **Fresh**

Berry: **Stylish**

Rose: **Romantic**

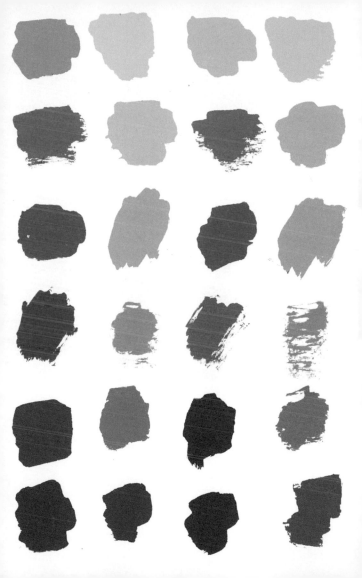

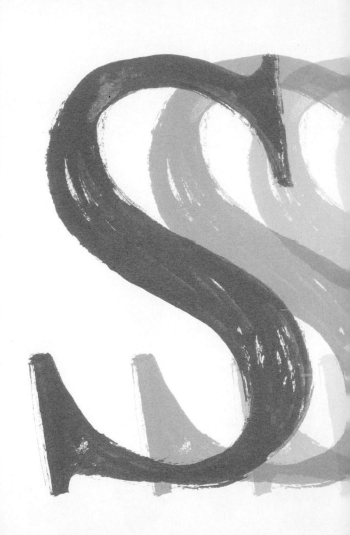

is for SHEER

If you're a total novice, sheer lipsticks are the way to ease into lip color. You'll need to reapply frequently to maintain the shade and shine you're looking for, but this will also help you learn to see how a simple swipe of lipstick lights up your face.

Lip tip: Sheer lipsticks are ideal for occasions when a bold dress or jewelry are making a strong statement, and you only want a hint of color on your lips.

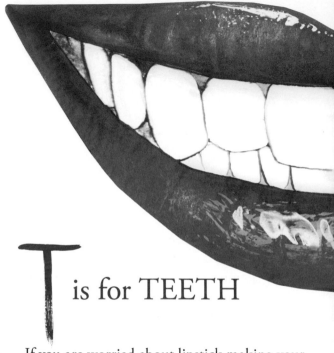

T is for TEETH

If you are worried about lipstick making your teeth look yellow, opt for blue-based cool colors (colors that tend to have some pink in them). The blue undertones will cut the yellow hue of the teeth and make your teeth look brighter.

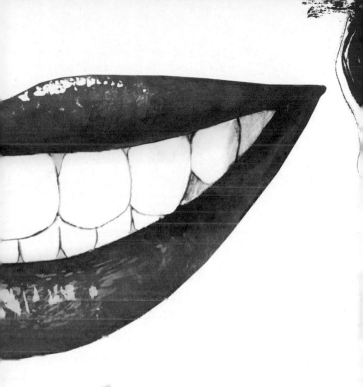

Lip tip: To prevent lipstick from getting on your teeth, after you apply, put your index finger in your mouth, pucker up, and then pull your finger through the lips. This removes all the lipstick on the inside of your mouth that could later get on your teeth.

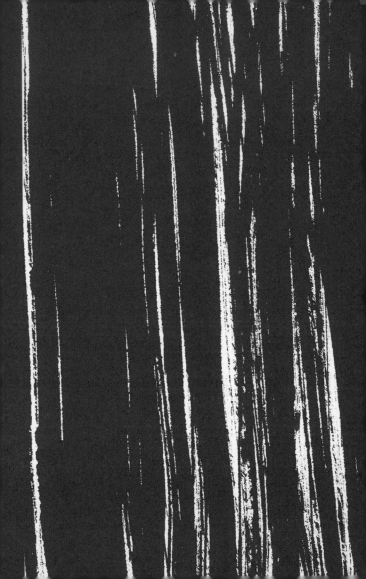

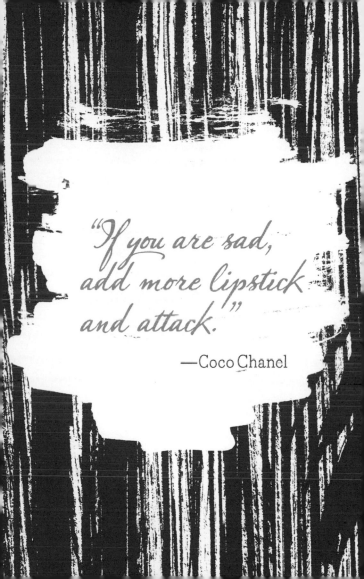

"If you are sad, add more lipstick and attack."

—Coco Chanel

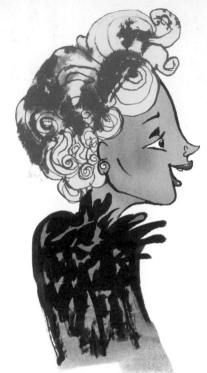

U is for UNEXPECTED

Unexpected things happen when you wear lipstick! People love to talk to you about the color you are wearing. You'll be surprised to see that a bold lip choice can be a real conversation starter that connects you to people.

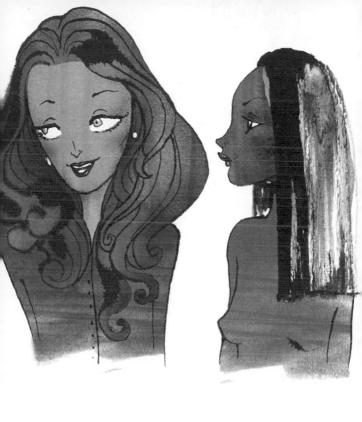

Lip tip: Try wearing the same shade of lipstick every day for a week and see how many people notice and comment on it—chances are, you will make new friends!

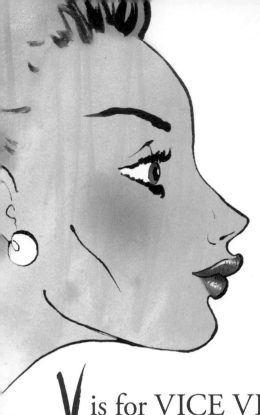

V is for VICE VERSA

Adopt the vice-versa principle for quick and easy cosmetics application. The bolder your lip color, the more minimal your eye makeup should be. And the more minimal your lips, the more dramatic you can be with your eyes.

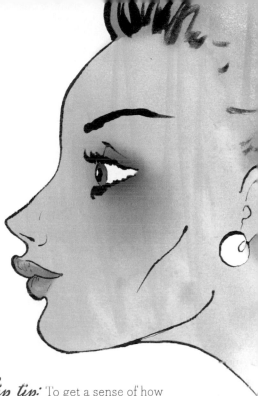

Lip tip: To get a sense of how bright or bold a lip color is, swipe it on the inside pad of your index finger. This is the best way to see what a hue will look like on your lips, as the skin there is closer to your natural lip color and texture than the skin on the back of your hand.

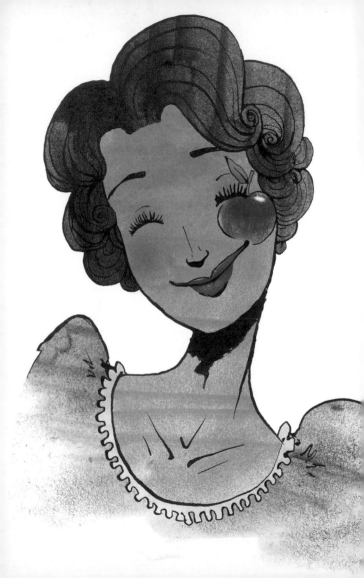

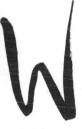

W is for WARMTH

Want to add warmth to your look, but don't have any blush on hand? Try this neat trick popular in the golden years of Hollywood. Dab the same lipstick you're using on your lips on the apples of your cheeks. You'll be amazed at how this one touch harmonizes your entire face.

> *Lip tip:* Smile wide—the roundest part of your cheek is the "apple."

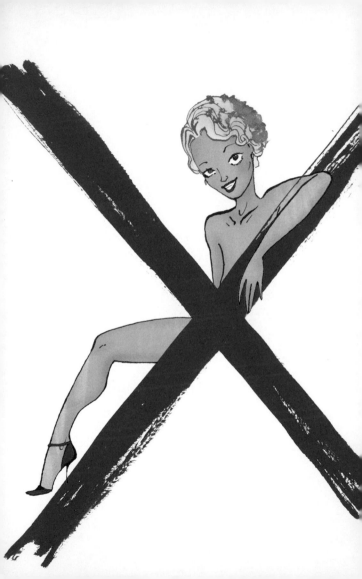

is for X FACTOR

Lipstick is fashion's X factor—the thing that can take a look from good to great in a heartbeat. It can be your X factor, too—the little thing that gives you an extra boost of confidence when you need it most.

Lip tip: Beauty is all about attitude: the most beautiful women are the ones who light up a room with their confidence and grace. Lipstick works the same way. Wear that lip color with aplomb—like you were born wearing it—and wait for the compliments to roll in.

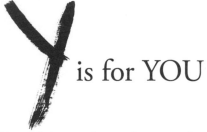

Y is for YOU

Lipstick is not about pleasing other people—it is about pleasing yourself. It helps you celebrate yourself and will encourage you to draw on the best of yourself from the inside out.

> *Lip tip:* Each time you apply your lipstick, reaffirm your commitment to being the best you can be on any given day. Some days that will feel easy, and other days that will be hard—but lipstick will always help.

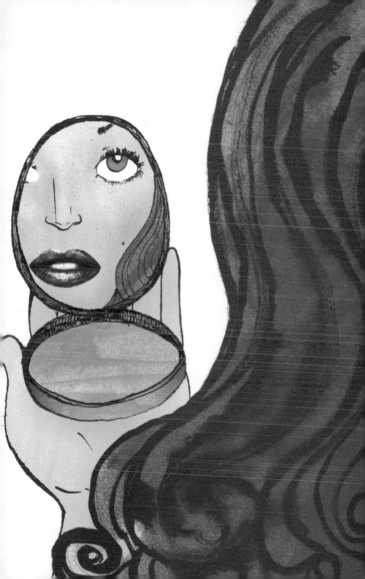

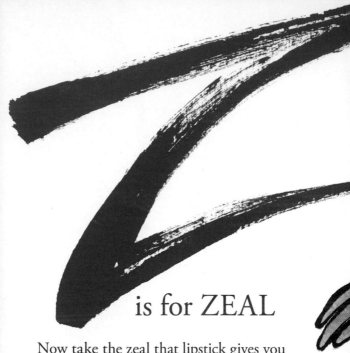

is for ZEAL

Now take the zeal that lipstick gives you
and apply it to everything you do. Lipstick
changed my life forever, and it could do the
same for you.

{ *Lip tip:* Whenever self-doubt
strikes, try a new lipstick!

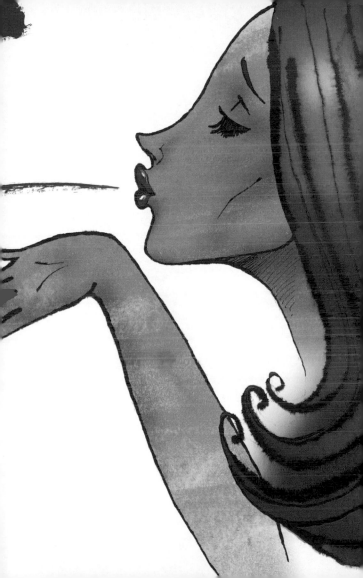

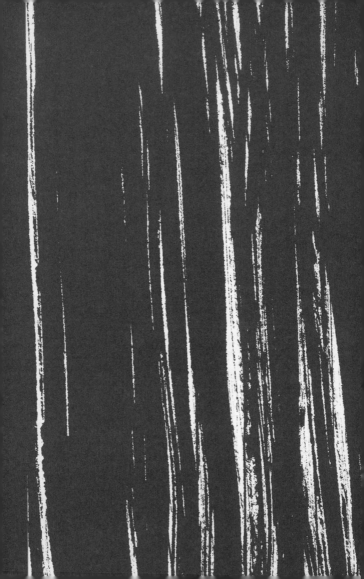

"Live your eyeliner, breathe your lipstick, and kill for each other."

—Lady Gaga

My Most Memorable Lipstick Moments

In my lifelong love affair with lipstick, there have been moments where it became far more than a cosmetic—moments that epitomized the connection lipstick can have to the deepest part of ourselves. Here are a few of mine.

1. My father died of cancer when I was seven years old. For months after, I wore a ballet tutu and red lipstick every day—a kind of mourning dress in reverse. Even at the age of seven, I sensed that channeling glamour would somehow protect me. It was the first time I saw lipstick as a way to help transcend sadness.

2. When I was around fourteen years old, my best friend and I were caught shoplifting lipsticks. We were at the local pharmacy after school, and we were in our uniforms when we concealed a few lipsticks in our sleeves. When we ran to catch the tram, the lipsticks

rolled out of our sleeves and down the hill in full view of a fellow student's mother. She identified us to the pharmacist, and a few days later we found ourselves back in his store, apologizing. "You'll never get anywhere with that behavior," he scolded us. He was right about the stealing but not about the risk taking: after all, going to all costs to get the lipstick I wanted eventually changed my life.

3. At the height of my teenage years the video that was playing everywhere was Robert Palmer's "Addicted to Love." In it, an army of beautiful, serious-looking girls wearing red lipstick and slicked-back hair flank him as he sings. It was at this time that my friends and I were going to nightclubs on the weekends, even though we were not yet of legal age. To fool the door person, we worked hard to look like we belonged. We never left home without our lipstick—it was always the final touch and completed our transformations from teenagers to adults. With my lipstick on, I had a vision of the type of woman I wanted to become: a powerful one.

4. At age nineteen, I drove to pick up the first production run of my very own lipstick. There were seven thousand lipsticks in total (seven shades and one thousand units a shade). I was piling them into the trunk of my old car (a car so old that it didn't even have a tape deck; instead, I kept a boom box in the front seat that I used to play Madonna's "Holiday"), when it dawned on me that I had literally *thousands* of lipsticks that I had no idea how to sell. But the challenge thrilled me, and I realized I was more afraid of not giving something a go than I was of failing. That belief has stuck with me ever since.

5. In 1995 I was awarded a very prestigious award: the Young Australian of the Year, which was given by the Prime Minister. It usually went to sports heroes. I was the first entrepreneur ever to receive it, and I was only twenty-three years old. Considering I had been expelled from a conservative school ten years before (because they told me I was too "different" and didn't fit in), it wasn't bad to be getting the highest honor

in the land. And all for lipstick. But of course, it wasn't *just* for lipstick: it was for what lipstick made me feel capable of.

6. I was not yet living in New York, but I happened to be in downtown Manhattan on the morning of September 11, 2001. It was the day that a city that felt so omnipotent suddenly became so vulnerable. Very quickly, a makeshift memorial sprung up in Union Square, because the city below Fourteenth Street was closed off to nonresidents. I went there and left one of my lipsticks as a symbol of defiance. The name of that lipstick happened to be Courage.

As you can see, courage is what lipstick has given me in every area of my life—it has always helped me access my own internal strength.

Whether it's a bright red lip or a daring new business venture, the only way you'll ever know if you can pull something off is if you try. I hope this book inspires you to be bold: in your lipstick *and*, more importantly, in your life.

Epilogue

What a difference the small things in life can make—whether it's getting lost in a good book, sharing a glass of wine with a dear friend, or livening up your look with a new lipstick. If nothing else, life is but a series of moments. One of the reasons I love lipstick is that applying it forces you to take a moment for yourself.

It's a moment that connects women all over the world—that moment in the mirror when we transcend the ordinary and reach for the extraordinary. I believe that lipstick more than any other cosmetic or fashion statement is deeply rooted in the power of the female psyche.

Somehow, there is magic in lipstick—and tapping into that magic makes the world a better place.

Just look at my story:

There once was a girl who felt blue
So what was that poor girl to do?
She knew what it was that she loved;
It was lipstick she treasured above.
In search of the right ones for her
She could only concur
That to find what she wanted
It was she who concocted
A company to make her dreams come true
And now she wants the same for you,
So go forth and try—
No more will you cry,
"I don't know what lipstick will do!"
For in the pages that have come before
You have found there is no single law.
Now you will see the change
That only a lipstick can arrange,
And before you know it, you too
Will be living each day anew—
With your lipstick on, this is just the beginni
Of happy, happy lipstick living!

Acknowledgments

I would like to acknowledge Fiona McCarthy—without you this book may never have happened. I would also like to acknowledge the wonderful Judith Curr and Sarah Cantin at Atria Books, and the incredibly talented David Foote: all of you have made this magical. Thank you as well to Dan Mandel, my agent, and to Stephanie Bonadio, who really encouraged me. And thank you to every single person who enjoys this book!